Acknowledgments

Firstly I would like to thank my wife and my children who have put up with me during these years of experiments and various fixations to lose weight.

Thanks to my friends at Babyluna who were the first to witness the success of my method.

Finally I would like to thank Samuele who gave me the support and help to return to a life of sport and well-being.

INDEX

Living to eat?

I was born in a town with the typical culture of southern Italy where the first thought when you wake up is "*what are we going to eat today*"? and even before finishing lunch the question is "*and what are we having for dinner*"?

My elderly parents were and are foodies and are excellent cooks. Obviously they have had to deal with their physical form since adolescence.

They are both obese. My father weighs 160 kg and my mother and sister both weigh 120 kg so they are in good company.

To better describe the scene, I remember that when my maternal grandfather, opened the door to me, at any time of the day I went there, immediately after greeting me, without my having spoken a single word yet, shouted loudly to my grandmother "*Pia !! give this child something to eat!*".

I cannot forget the Sunday lunches we were invited to. The table was laden with food for 30 people when only 10 people were invited. There had to be leftovers for them to be satisfied.

The fate of the obese was already written in my genetic heritage.

At the age of 10 my nickname was *spray can* because of my body shape. In the summer between the end of elementary school and the beginning of middle school I was 11, and a sort of miracle happened. I was going to a new school, new environment, new friends (or enemies) in September, and realized that I had to do something to change my reputation, especially with girls.

That was my first adolescent stimulus, and it was very strong.

That summer I started doing sports every day. I will never forget that my family had ice cream with fresh cream (the best in town) every night and I abstained as if I had made a vow even though my mother tried to tempt me saying "*but at least taste a bit*".

I had the determination and tenacity of a Tibetan monk and couldn't understand where all this strength came from because I actually wanted to eat everything in the ice cream shop.

The fact is that I was beginning to see the first results, my waistline was smaller, I needed new clothes, I managed to tie my shoe laces more easily and my peers approved and no longer classified me in the fat category.

Social approval was a strong motivation to continue.

As I grew up I increased my sporting activity so much that I could eat as much as 5 people and always stayed in shape. No joke.

I set my record in a basketball camp where there were so many spoiled little children who ate very little and systematically left all sorts of goodies on the plates. To me it was like the restaurants on the big cruise ships, you could eat as much as you liked. The "*all you can eat*" formula.

I already had the fixation of not wasting and throwing away food by virtue of a sort of moral principle against poverty in the world that was instilled in me from an early age.

I made friends with some of the most squeamish kids, who sat next to me and arranged for them to sneak their plates of food to me (practically intact) and I literally made their contents disappear.

They weren't scolded by the coach who assured the unsuspecting parents that their children ate up everything. I will never forget that in addition to my food, I managed to swallow 5 first courses, 4 main dishes and 18 slices of pineapple.

I really deserved the nickname "vacuum cleaner", but I was fine and in good shape.

After the age of 23, my weight fluctuated ranging from an increase of 10 kg up to more than 20 kg around the age of 30 depending on my indulgences.

During my university years I lived in various highly populated communities and there was always a good reason to celebrate and to celebrate meant to eat everything from appetizers to desserts, including drinks. I began to drink wine, alcohol, coffee (always with sugar) and to eat all kinds of cakes and desserts almost every day. I went from being overweight to being obese. I had put on 40 kg. I was almost unrecognizable from the time I ran around the basketball fields.

I got engaged and then decided to get married. I had to fit into my suit so I lost a few kilos. For a while after the wedding I was careful about what I ate but soon after I went back to my old habits.

It was shocking how easy it was to put on weight and how difficult it was to lose weight. A harsh law of nature.

Thus from the 20-year weight of 78 kg I reached 118 kg.

The funny and ridiculous thing was that if I looked at myself in the mirror I always saw the same thing, that is, my mind didn't see the differences and I felt almost like I was thin. I was convinced that the weight increase was due to muscle mass.

At one point, while the boat of will and health was completely adrift, my wife, like a bolt from the blue, screamed "*if you don't lose weight I'll leave you*".

They were the early years of marriage and I still loved her enough to find the time and the desire to consult a nutritionist. Or at least pretend that I was interested in doing so.

There was a solution. I contacted an old friend with the intention of having a "free" consultation with regards the quantity of food that should be eaten.

I went to see her with the excuse that it was my father who needed advice, and it was true because even my old man had exceeded certain limits, and so at the end of the visit, I casually asked her if she could also write a magic formula for me. A diet.

My father and I followed the diet for about 10 months.

Obviously I followed the diet much less seriously than my father, but I needed a plausible justification to make my wife understand that I was trying and that I cared for her.

I still managed to lose 15 kg while my father who was more serious and reliable than me, lost 26kg.

Those results were thwarted after a few months, both by my father and I.

It is the dramatic but inexorable "yo-yo" or "accordion" effect of diets that after an initial enthusiasm make you put on the kilos lost with interest. Later I will explain to you why this phenomenon almost always occurs.

I then said, that's enough, I would not follow any other "diet", after all my life was fine for what I had to do. I didn't have to please anyone, and my wife, a mother of three, would have understood.

It was obvious that I was not stimulated. For what reasons or for whom should I have been subjected to stress and deprivation? Eating is one of the pleasures of life. My motto was "*I don't want to live like a sick man to then die a healthy man*".

However, I went from one fixation to another, I confess that I have never missed them. Every obsession was justified by a pseudo scientific foundation that in my opinion was always a kind of revolution and the remedy for every problem for my obesity.

At one stage I drank large quantities of green tea and I only ate rice. I put lemon on everything and ate very small meals 10 times a day, then I switched to alkaline thinking and integral carbohydrates and finally to fast walks.

They are good, I said, they do not cause trauma to the joints and they make you lose weight. The last fixation was water with baking soda. I drank more water than a camel before crossing the desert.

My weight however was the only thing that remained constant and showed no signs of changing while fixations came and went. None of them worked. Was I still alive?

Yes, of course. Food remained an indispensable pleasure for me. I lived to eat food in a completely disorderly manner.

At the age of 45 weighing 118 kg and 183 cm in height, while I was attending a basketball training session for my son, a dear friend sat next to me and said *"you were good, why you don't play again*?".

The question flattered me and he reminded me of the good old days when I managed to hit the basket and the opponents couldn't beat me. I replied no thank you, you are kind but I can't, I'm completely out of shape and I don't want to play again. I knew that I would only make a fool of myself and would end up playing like a fool in the middle of the field.

That question, however, echoed in my mind several times and, after a few days, it became the umpteenth non-food fixation, or rather, a sort of challenge to my pride.

I said to myself, why not? With a little commitment I could start playing like before and I could even lose weight.

A fantasy that almost became reality. I remember the first training session.

After 2 minutes I had to throw myself to the ground like a dead weight, my heart was beating like never before, everything was misty and my head was spinning. I thought it was normal; after all it was the first training session after so many years. I did not attribute the sick feeling to my weight.

However, my condition did not improve even after other training sessions. I was convinced that sooner or later I would lose weight. I drank a lot of water and sometimes fasted in the evening. Obviously to no avail.

By pure chance one day, on accompanying my father to the cardiologist, I decided to talk to him about the tachycardia.

After asking me a few questions he told me that it could be caused by the malfunctioning of my thyroid gland so he advised me to have a check up. One of my friends who is a radiologist did an ultrasound on my neck. Oh dear, there were many micro nodules. Hashimoto's thyroiditis.

It is a well known fact that men, unlike women, complain when they have fever at 37 degrees. So for a time before consulting the very gracious endocrinologist, I thought my end was near. And I was serious. I almost made a will.

In a week of studying doctor's opinions and self-styled more or less enlightened scientists intensely on the web, who explained everything about the thyroid.

What it is, how it works, why it decomposes and, above all, what one must and mustn't do. The more information I got the more anxious I became.

There are different theories, but everyone agreed on the importance of good nutrition and a good lifestyle.

I had blood tests and specialist examinations. It was clear that my situation was common to that of many other people and that there was nothing serious that could not be resolved, but, and here comes the best part, the pretty specialist categorically ordered me to lose weight and say goodbye to obesity (118 kg).

Here we go again. Another diet !

This time I had a different stimulus, the need to be healthy. My life and my loved ones and everything I loved to do were worth the effort.

But in life one must be ready to make necessity a virtue and that was what I wanted to do this time as well. I've always been a free spirit and I've never liked strict methods.

I have never liked dieticians because they make you weigh your food, they make you count calories, and they ask you *"what job do you do? Do you practice any sport? ... then you must not eat more than 1500 calories a day "*.

No, they can't make me obey those rules.

I absolutely had to find someone who would tailor an eating plan for me, without giving me too many rules.

So I returned to my friend who this time I caught by surprise in her rooms when I entered between patients and, while she was sitting and looking at me from behind her desk, while standing in front of her, I asked, smiling. *"Please tell me what to eat to lose weight … I need just a little of your time"*. I had a recycled A4 sheet and a pen that barely wrote. It was a late morning in January and you could see the clear sky from the window.

She began to explain the criteria to be followed during daily meals, the preferred foods and what one can eat together and others to avoid. Stop. Thanks Jo. "*Let me know? I will see you again in a months' time*

In normal cases her patients visits lasted about an hour, I left her room after just 10 minutes with a piece of recycled paper in my hand with hurriedly written notes done while standing up.

However, before persuading myself to start this journey, I watched dozens of tutorials, weight-loss gurus, dieticians and all kinds of nutritional advice on *YouTube*.

Pills and magical foods, infallible and balanced healthy food products, that are compatible with our DNA.

I listened and watched everything like supporters of the Mediterranean diet, the Ketogenic and Palaeolithic Diets. There are various types of extremism.

And obviously, last but not least, my wife's advice was essential. An excellent cook (In my opinion a star chef) who systematically rejected everything I had learned here and there, including my friend's criteria.

In the end you will put together all the information you have by making a personal summary. It was the month of January.

After not even 5 months, in May, I had already lost 10 kg. As the weeks went by I could not believe my eyes, enthusiasm had the upper hand and people told me they were surprised that I had lost weight.

A wonderful feeling, but I did not succumb to the temptation of weighing myself every day. Every Tuesday morning, on an empty stomach, my electronic scale registered a lower figure than the previous week.

Sometimes there was no change, but my friend reassured me that it was normal. Weight loss is not always measured by a scale but rather by measuring the waistline. In fact you begin to lose fat mass, but the lean mass increases (muscles) and therefore even if the scale shows the same weight you feel that your jeans are looser. However, every 500 g loss was a victory for me and an incentive to continue.

Each time I weighed myself I took a picture of the number with my smart phone and all week I looked at it to convince myself it was real and to make comparisons over time.

The best thing is that even today, after more than a year, I have not had the yo-yo effect and I manage to stay in shape without making special sacrifices. I swear I never weighed anything apart from carbohydrates and I can proudly say that I follow no "diet", but I have certainly changed my eating style and especially my lifestyle.

I think that I have found the right direction for myself.

I want to show you the path that I followed because I am absolutely convinced that if I have succeeded, it is possible for anyone to succeed.

This obviously excludes the cases of particular pathologies that require prescriptions from a specialist doctor. I believe there is a direction for everyone; we just need to get ourselves a compass or a method to orient ourselves and not get lost.

Before revealing in detail what, how much and how I eat during the day and throughout the week, I want to try to convey concepts that I consider very important because they have changed the way I see things and interact with food.

It is important to know why diets do not work, understand what basal metabolism is and how it accelerates, appreciate the fundamental role of proteins, choose which type of physical activity to do and finally I will give you the food criteria I followed.

All diets fail ... sooner or later

My parents have tried many "diets" over the years, every year a new one comes out based on the current fashion, it seemed to be the decisive or scientifically safest one.

They have remained obese like so many people I know.

There is a huge amount of information on the web.

There are constantly new proposals, books, scientific studies that guarantee lasting results at a good price.

However, after a short period of enthusiasm, 90% of cases fail over and over again. The current diets sell you the illusion of fixing your eating mistakes and changing your body to look like a Hollywood star in a short time.

In fact, if you follow a diet where you drastically reduce calories without associating physical activity to increase muscle mass, you will lose weight in the beginning because you will lose both fat and lean mass (muscles), but your metabolism will slow down at the same pace until the weight loss stops.

It is only at this stage that certain dieticians tell you that you have to "unlock" your metabolism, but actually, the yo-yo effect is a moment, with the aggravating circumstance that, having slowed further the basal metabolism (which I will explain soon), your body will no longer burn calories like before and the consequence is that you will recover the lost kilos with very high interest. I have personally proven that there is no standard diet suitable for everyone and forever and that the approach to counting calories is only a partial aspect and not the most important factor for change that needs to be customized. We are all individuals and are all very different from each other.

This is why I realized that it is wrong to follow a diet. Change is and must be gradual and starts from our heads.

Your mental state, that is the belief that you have to do something to change your state of non-wellbeing, is the first step to change your lifestyle. Your determination has a fundamental role. This is why you need a valid stimulus.

Above all you have to ask yourself and answer if it is really necessary for you to change your lifestyle?

Then you have to ask yourself why you should change? And finally you have to ask yourself if you can do it alone? The answer is no, but in a sense, yes.

No because you need someone or something that supports you and gives you a reason to do it, yes because you have to make that reason your own, it must grow and take shape within you.

You must be convinced, otherwise I advise you not to do anything, stay just as you are because after the enthusiasm of the first kilos lost, you will inevitably return to a worse state than the one you started with, with the aggravating circumstance of having experienced, for the umpteenth time, the disappointment of not having achieved a goal that seemed within reach. You will be convinced once again that you won't be able to do it and that diets are not for you. Until once again you consult the Guru of the moment who will tell you about a new formula or magic pill, to continue to fail and follow the vicious circle of failures.

When we refer to a "*diet*" we think it is something temporary, linked for example to the bathing costume test, the event of the year to wear a certain type of dress, your child's wedding or your friend's university degree party.

We believe that a diet consists of depriving ourselves of food, of making sacrifices, of spending time cooking, eating salad and wasting time shopping.

I often meet people who repeat *"I have been on diet all my life"* and in fact I have never noticed a change in their waistline. I sincerely hope that at the end of reading this book you can understand that starting is not complicated and continuing is even easier if you begin to see your goal on the horizon.

Increase your metabolism

What I am going to tell you now is of fundamental importance because the revolution of my lifestyle started from this understanding.

Have you ever heard someone complaining or have you ever complained about "*I have a slow metabolism*" or "*there is something that slows down my calorie consumption*". I would say you have, and you have often associated it with the concept of "*I have to do more exercise*" or "*I sit too much*".

First of all it is true that the state of our body largely depends on whether our metabolism functions well or not. What is metabolism? We can say briefly that it is the combination of biochemical reactions like the catabolic reactions that consume energy in the tissues to produce work and the anabolic ones that reconstruct the tissues.

I don't want to go into specific medical terms, but the balance of these two branches of metabolism characterizes the state of your body.

As long as you are growing and are young, you tend to stay in an anabolic position which switches to the catabolic one as you get older. In the case of body mass regulation, when your metabolism slows down, you have difficulty burning calories and increase fat storage. Surely there is the factor of the ratio between calories eaten and consumed, but there are also many other aspects that nobody has ever told you about.

The fundamental question is: what does my "energy expenditure" depend on the quantity of calories I consume? The answer will shock you.

It is a fact that around 60% of the calories consumed depends on the basal metabolism, or rather on what you consume simply to stay alive and while resting. 20-30% depends on physical activity, or active consumption of calories, and finally for the remaining part on the thermogenic effect of foods, that is, on how many calories you have to consume to metabolize the foods you eat.

These are the factors that determine the overall energy consumption in a person.

As you can see, the highest percentage of consumption concerns the basal metabolic rate (60%).

Yes, you understood correctly, what your body consumes without moving. An analogy can be made by comparing the basal metabolic rate to the cylinder capacity of a car. With the same fuel (calories) a car with a higher cylinder capacity (for example a SUV) will consume more than a small car with a lower cylinder capacity engine. The same amount of fuel will end sooner and will be "burned" by the SUV more than by the smaller vehicle.

In the same way, two subjects with different basal metabolism functioning, who eat the same foods and consume the same calories will develop different consumptions: the person with a faster and more efficient basal metabolism will burn more calories than those with a slower basal metabolism, simply standing still and doing nothing.

You may have observed, and perhaps felt a little jealous, to see that there are people who eat an enormous amount without gaining a gram, while you gain weight just by breathing.

Here, the difference lies in having a different basal metabolism. If 60% of energy consumption depends on the basal metabolic rate, you understand that it is not worth focusing on what has a lower impact such as physical activity which accounts for about 20-30% of energy consumption. This certainly is important but only if done in a certain way that I will explain later.

So you ask, can I increase the capacity of my engine? Can I increase my basal metabolism and therefore energy consumption? The answer is yes, you can.

Well, first of all your engine capacity depends on your muscle mass. The more efficient muscle you have, the more you will consume simply by standing still. The less efficient muscles you have, the fewer calories you will burn, and the harder it will be to maintain the correct amount of fat, unless you drastically reduce the intake of calories, which leads to the risk of a further loss of muscle mass. It's a vicious cycle, but at the same time virtuous if we exploit it properly. To reactivate the metabolism means to focus on maintaining and reconstructing muscle mass. You don't have to become a young Arnold Schwarzenegger, in fact it is sufficient to make the muscular system, which has fallen asleep due to the wrong lifestyle, take on tone. Great.

Do you understand? Then you will think, if so, it is so easy, I will join a gym, increase my muscle mass and lose weight automatically.

You could have given this information by writing two sentences instead of writing a book. As you will discover later, the increase in muscle mass not associated with balanced eating is not enough.

Your basal metabolism will definitely increase but this alone will not promote weight loss and the existing fat will be added to the muscle weight therefore your scale will show an increase rather than a decrease in weight.

We must give our body the right intake of macronutrients such as fibre, carbohydrates, fats and above all proteins that the muscles largely feed on.

Proteins

That we need to practice proper nutrition is intuitive as is the fact that we must practice adequate and constant work outs. However, not everyone knows that proteins more than all foods allow an increase in muscle mass and that, due to their assimilation, they need a greater consumption of calories compared to other nutrients, thus offering an additional thermogenic advantage.

So by eating proteins, you do two things, nourish and increase the power of the "cylinders" of your engine and benefit from the thermogenic advantage, which means you consume more calories to assimilate them. You therefore understand that correct protein consumption combined with certain physical activity (I will explain later) is the first step to reactivate the metabolism.

The classic approach of working out more, reducing caloric intake by penalizing proteins in favour of carbohydrates is not the right thing to do. If you are doing it, change your lifestyle and change direction. And if you are penalizing proteins you will not be able to benefit from the thermogenic effect of this important macro nutrient.

Today negative thoughts are often linked to proteins, especially those derived from animals. I don't want to discriminate or judge vegetarians, vegans or other eating habits, but it is clear that we need to ask ourselves what animal proteins we are talking about and try to eat as much biological food as possible. In particular, I want to talk about a super-protein food that I started eating every day and that contributed to improving my well-being.

Eggs.

Lots of negative things have been said about eggs, for years it seemed that they were to be avoided and that they even did more harm than a hot dog. The recommendation *"be careful not to eat too many eggs"* has no scientific basis.

Eggs are a super healthy food.

It is true that they contain cholesterol, but eating food that contains cholesterol is not the same as having high cholesterol in the body, they are two distinct things.

The cholesterol that is measured by a blood test, is largely the cholesterol produced by the liver and is not directly related to cholesterol in food. The hepatic production of cholesterol is stimulated by many factors, for example refined grains (white flours) and sugars.

Regular consumption of eggs increases HDL which is the good component of cholesterol that cleans the arteries. In 30% of cases there is also an increase in LDL in a benign form. So eggs do not have contraindications for cholesterol. Not only that, but eggs have excellent biological proteins and contain many other nutrients that are important, such as carotenoids, vitamins, omega 3 or fatty acids that are anti-inflammatory, especially if they are organic products. However, it is always important to understand in what nutritional context they are consumed.

If, in fact, we eat half a kilo of bacon and a slice of cream cake, the beneficial effect of this super food vanishes. This is to make you understand that healthy foods should not be isolated and should be contextualized in a balanced diet.

When we talk about balanced nutrition, we must also pay attention to food associations and quantities.

For example, if you eat lots of eggs all at once it is not good for you just because eggs are a healthy food. Likewise, it is not a good idea to combine many healthy foods together; on the contrary it can be a harmful chemical mixture. And yet, the effect of the intake of good fats in a diet rich in sugars is different and produces negative effects compared to the intake of fats in the absence of sugars. This is why we must never isolate different types of food but consider them in a global context.

Fats are important and should not be reduced but selected, choosing the healthy ones. In conclusion you can eat one or two eggs every day, especially for breakfast if you work out for muscle growth.

What physical activity should you do?

There is often a lot of confusion when it comes to what physical exercise to do to lose weight.

Restoring sufficient and adequate muscle tone to reactivate the basal metabolism does not mean doing just any activity, especially if it is "aerobic" like running, cycling, fast walks or all activities that last for an average or long time.

Now I am going to amaze you again.

You have always thought that by doing lots of activities that make you sweat, which means more aerobic activity, you can achieve greater results in terms of weight loss.

I remember the scene of a guy who was running with a kind of plastic bag wrapped around his abdominal area under the scorching sun, believing that he would lose more weight because he was sweating more in that painful area of his body. Today I smile at the thought of it.

Aerobic training is certainly good for the heart and lungs, but if it is prolonged it causes you to lose lean mass, which is muscle mass, that slows down the basal metabolism.

You can lose weight, of course, but be aware that you are not decreasing the fat mass, but the lean mass (the muscles). Exercising is very important but it does not have a big impact on the energy expenditure of the person if you do not include muscular type exercises (anaerobic) that will allow you to increase your basal metabolism to achieve a big impact on the regulation of body weight and the fat percentage.

Let's clarify that when we talk about physical activity it is better to use the term training. The difference is important, because training means planning objectives and means to reach these objectives and measure the results gradually.

This undoubtedly requires constancy and regularity. Instead physical activity in the generic sense is something that can be done even sporadically, like a walk in the park or a game with friends when the weather is good.

But it is not the right way to increase muscle mass.

As I said, you don't have to become a body builder. Muscle is much more than something to show off, it is important for every daily action, like picking up shopping bags from the ground, holding children in your arms, lowering yourselves and getting out of bed, getting off a sofa or a chair.

Often even these simple movements can become tiring or even cause injuries. This principle also applies in the case of very thin people without fat mass but with equally scarce or inefficient muscle mass.

It is natural that as we grow older we become flabbier and that muscle tissue decreases in favour of fatty tissue, which is why sometimes body weight does not change but body composition changes: more fat mass and less lean mass.

You will feel more tired and you will not want to do anything, except always look for a chair to sit on or a sofa to lie on. Muscles respond well according to how we move and the stimuli we create for them. If we run a long distance we create an elongated musculature that is different from if we run in sprint mode, with short strides.

Thus the muscle adapts to the loads to which we subject it and it activates different energy metabolism mechanisms that have different consequences on anatomical, endocrine and metabolic levels.

To increase the basal metabolic rate it is sufficient to stimulate the muscle with an adequate load to generate a hypertrophic response, the muscle must be forced to pick up the load, to the extent that it suffers and is damaged so it will be induced to create more structures and more mass.

This process should also be done gradually; you cannot start with excessive weights. You must first awaken and tone your muscles and gradually increase the load up to a certain limit, without exaggeration. At least three sessions a week are enough. I said enough but if you train every day it won't hurt you but you will have to diversify and maybe focus on different muscles every time. I'm not going to explain to you how you have to do a training session, but we all know that there is a first phase called warming up.

You can't start doing "cold" efforts. As soon as you have warmed up enough which is ideal for increasing muscle mass you need to do H.I.T. (height intensity training), that is short high intensity repetitions, rather than doing many long repetitions of the exercises. If this is done well, 20 minutes per day of HIT will suffice. The choice of time depends on many factors and each person will have to personalize and find their own ideal space in the organization of their day.

The most common training choice is machine weights.

It is an effective but not a functional system because the muscle acts in an isolated manner that is to say for the type of movement for which the machine is set. Our body and our daily actions require the synergic activation of muscle chains, that is, more muscles. These do not move and never act individually in anything we do. Think about it. When we lower ourselves to pick up the shopping bags, we activate not only the biceps, but also the leg, back and shoulder muscles.

Then there is cross fit and functional gymnastics with the use of kettle bells. Increasing the functional performance of the stimulated organism is overall a much more valid tool but if done at certain levels it can be difficult after a certain age. It could in fact cause injuries to the skeletal system especially if the exercises are not done correctly or the weights are excessive.

Finally, there is free body exercise which is an excellent idea for training, but if the exercises are not done according to the correct technique, sufficient loads are not generated to increase the muscular system. So the technical component can be an obstacle to many people starting from scratch.

Which method should you choose? Everyone must find the right solution for themselves. The result remains the same: to tone and increase muscle mass efficiently.

Personally I have experimented and refined a method that I consider to be innovative because it follows the principle of gradualness and can also be adapted to those starting from scratch in just one square meter of space, comfortably at home.

I usually work out in the morning soon after I wake up or in the evening before dinner. I do 20 minutes of HIT alternating exercises with light and heavier weights and free body exercises, with very short intervals of 10 seconds each. After training I have a shower that starts with hot water but ends with cold water. I have managed to resist for 3 minutes under the shower doing this.

I'll explain the reasons further on.

Starting the day with a cold shower has several physical and psychological health benefits. You can't imagine how many there are, even though the thought alone doesn't seem like a pleasant habit.

Of course, it may seem like torture but if you succeed, you are gradually taking control of the situation and telling yourself that you are ready to face whatever the day has in store for you. It really helps to strengthen your will power.

When cold water hits the skin, the natural reaction is to breathe much more deeply than usual. This increases the oxygen intake and speeds up circulation. Blood travels faster to limbs and organs, and improves brain function.

It therefore stimulates breathing, which decreases the Co2 levels in the body helping you to reduce stress levels and increase the immune response to stimulate white blood cells. According to research by the University of Maastricht, regular exposure to low temperatures helps to lose up to 4 pounds every year.

Part of the fat in our body is actually composed of brown fat cells which, if exposed to a cold situation, burn calories to warm the body up.

All athletes know that there is nothing more regenerating than an ice bath to solve muscle problems. The initial water flow blocks peripheral circulation and directs blood to the key organs. When it is no longer cold, the blood flows to the periphery, but is richer in oxygen. In this manner the tissues repair faster and the metabolism accelerates.

A hot shower seems to be the most relaxing thing for the skin. In fact this is not true, while hot water destroys the natural oil in the skin (using bubble bath only worsens the situation) cold water is much more delicate on the skin and tends to dry it out less.

Even more important than the superficial effects, however, the blood level is important: in fact, under a jet of cold water, the surface of the blood vessels narrows, causing the skin pores to close. Finally, washing hair with cold water makes it stronger and much shinier. Good blood flow also stimulates faster hair growth. It is a simple habit that, once it becomes second nature, is not terrifying at all.

Actually a final cold rinse is enough, without having to submit to the torture of a complete cold shower. Returning to training, you will know that you are on the right path only if you have some positive signals like being aware of feeling stronger and more energetic.

You will understand that you are training well and you are in the right direction only if you have some positive signals such as feeling stronger and more energetic.

If you feel weaker than before, then there is something wrong. You should be more resistant, be in a good mood, and catch less colds and flu. Those are signs that your immune system is getting stronger. Finally you must sleep well, not too little and not too much.

My food week

We have arrived at the last chapter of this journey.

Don't think that it is the most important thing because the path to success is a result of the combination of two essential factors, nutrition and physical activity.

Only nutrition or physical activity alone is not enough. I assure you that my dietary approach combined with targeted training, beyond the theories of any diet, has worked. I managed to lose weight and stay in shape without making special sacrifices, without weighing what I ate (apart from carbohydrates) and food is still one of the pleasures of my life.

The most important fact was and is to maintain a renewed state of global well-being.

There are no miracle foods but it is true that some foods in the context of healthy nutrition can help to lose fat but the effects that foods have on our body are not always the same and should not be evaluated only on the basis of the number of calories.

We must eat healthy foods that are not always perceived as such.

Let's start with the morning, a fundamental moment because it defines the tone of the day. Before telling you what I eat for breakfast, let me share some useful information because if we learn to manage the first moments of the day on a mental level, this translates into a great day and a great life. Don't grumble, a baby doesn't snort when it comes to light, but breathes.

The morning is the birth of a new day. If possible open a window and take a deep breath. Appreciate your life and be happy that you are alive. Don't take your life for granted.

Smile. Look in the mirror and admire yourself. Things that stimulate you from the outside change your emotional state. Everything starts within oneself.

Do not complain. We cannot always control external events, but we can manage internal events and change our interpretation of negative external events.

Before eating, drink at least one or two glasses of water. Always do this before every meal.

Consider water as your best friend.

There is an important study by the Japanese scientist Masaru Emoto that makes us understand why water is "alive". It carries information, we are made of water, and the world is made of water, without water we could not live.

Water is essential for our health and it is really good to drink it as soon as you wake up, it helps fight stomach acid, eliminate toxins, purify the kidneys, improve circulation and prevent constipation.

For some people, eating in the morning is a sore point and many skip breakfast, not because they are applying the technique of intermittent fasting and are voluntarily controlling their food intake by skipping a meal, but because they are in a hurry or simply don't feel hungry.

This habit has negative repercussions during the day because it is as if you have left with the engine flooded without energy. You will look for food compensations later and find it in harmful foods. The best thing to do is to change your habits.

The majority of people who have breakfast choose a sweet breakfast. Sugars however, are foods that, even in a context of a correct caloric balance, are unfavourable because they affect the metabolism negatively and make fat loss more difficult. This is because they cause a hyper production of insulin that does not facilitate loss but favours the accumulation of fat, especially abdominal fat.

It is therefore necessary to change from a sweet breakfast to one which is rich in nutrients with a lower glycemic load and make it a more complete meal.

Here is a list of beneficial foods for this purpose: eggs, fresh seasonal fruit, avocado, walnut or almond cream (obviously unsweetened), whole grains, almond milk, oatmeal, rice, green tea and plain yogurt.

Of course without adding sugar and a maximum of two or three teaspoons of honey. You don't have to eat them all of course. Make a selection of those that have the three fundamental quotas, the protein, fibre and carbohydrates quota. These three parts must always be included in every meal. Even these days the so-called "dissociated diet" is in fashion, that is, to divide carbohydrates from proteins. Carbohydrates are usually eaten for lunch and proteins in the evening.

Meals must always be complete but balanced.

Of course carbohydrates should be avoided in the evening excluding potatoes.

A fibre portion should always prevail in every meal, while the protein and carbohydrate portions should be the same. Personally I always follow this ritual at breakfast: a seasonal fruit, peanut butter (no more than 3 teaspoons), an egg, and two slices of wholemeal bread or 4 whole-wheat rusks and a little bit of sugar-free yogurt.

Every so often I add a few teaspoons of organic honey of which I know the origins. In some countries industrial honey is often adulterated. In fact, honey is counterfeited using different varieties of syrup, rice or diluted with sugar syrup. In the middle of the morning, if I'm hungry, I eat some dried fruit, like almonds, walnuts or seeds.

The supermarkets sell packets with excellent mixes.

I now drink coffee without sugar. It's just a matter of habit, and you will eventually like the taste. At lunch I prefer to eat one dish with raw vegetables (no tomatoes), not more than 80 grams of wholegrain cereals (brown, black or red rice, quinoa, pasta or whole-wheat bread), rotating proteins (white meat, red meat and eggs). I advise you not to consume more than 400 g of red meat per week. In the afternoon if I am hungry I make a snack based on fresh seasonal fruit.

I always have cooked or grilled vegetables for dinner unlike at lunchtime. I have a portion of protein like fish or vegetables in rotation which is always different to what I had at lunch. As I have mentioned, no carbohydrates should be eaten in the evening, except for potatoes, preferably sweet potatoes (200 grams maximum), especially if I have done physical exercise in the afternoon.

Vegetables should not be considered as a simple side dish, 50% of lunch and dinner should ideally consist of vegetables, and the other 50% should be 25% of cereals and 25% of proteins.

You can decide the rotation of the combinations during the week; you can change the order without changing the result. It is clear that you will have to shop differently. I advise you to plan your menu for the whole week. Personally, I consider it a waste of time to go shopping every day.

These are only qualitative, quantitative and associative criteria.

I can assure you that today I eat more than when I was obese and I am absolutely never hungry. As already mentioned, but I don't take it for granted, you shouldn't overdo it even if the food is healthy. I can't eat a "healthy" calf or pig just because they are proteins. By "healthy" we mean not only the quality of the food, but also the context in which we eat it and therefore the associations with other macronutrients.

If any good food or even water is consumed in exaggeration it is harmful.

I believe that generally the secret consists of knowing how to balance and combine fundamental macro-foods, proteins, carbohydrates and fats.

Fats can be used if they are good products such as extra virgin olive oil or unsaturated fats in dried fruit. Today, after almost 50 years of condemning fats, science agrees that fats are not bad for you when eaten in a healthy diet.

Also the use of salt must be limited but not completely eliminated unless your doctor specifically prescribes it for a particular reason. Everyone must personalize their eating habits to suit themselves using common sense and above all, if you have health problems or food intolerances, consult a specialist.

Forget about French fries, sausages, inappropriate condiments, certain industrial products made and designed to be irresistible and addictive. Forget about desserts and everything that contains sugar. The body gets sugar from vegetables, fruit and whole grains. Drink very little alcohol and avoid it if you can. A maximum of half a glass of alcohol per meal is acceptable.

Eating well sometimes costs a little more, but staying healthy is priceless.

It's better to spend a little more to eat healthier than to buy medicine and pay for treatment.

Here is a final general indication on how to eat food.

First of all, I advise you to always sit down when you eat rather than walk around or stand. Chew a lot and slowly, don't swallow too much in rotation, like in the cartoons.

Never eat from packets, take at least three deep breaths before starting to eat to activate the parasympathetic and sympathetic nervous system.

And if I'm out with friends or there is a party must I be antisocial and wave a flag saying that I am changing my lifestyle? A plausible question, the answer to which is no, never be antisocial.

One or two unscheduled meals per week are acceptable and should not make you feel guilty. You will soon start to eat in a balanced way again compensating by avoiding carbohydrates the next day and eating only vegetables and proteins.

Seeing one swallow does not mean that it is spring.

Bit by bit you will realize that you will tend to reject wrong food because you are following a different lifestyle. Be careful not to fast after an unscheduled program, it serves no purpose except to damage your metabolism and does more harm than good. When you binge, in the evening eat only vegetables even if you are not hungry. Today it is fashionable to talk about intermittent fasting that probably has some foundation but also negative points. In fact the metabolic response to fasting in sensitive people can raise the level of cortisol, so it is not said that it is good for everyone or that it is always a success.

Fasting is a kind of alarm bell for the organism and is perceived as a potential danger that the metabolism translates into the signal *"hold the fat that there is"* and it is the same signal that develops when a person is very stressed. This is why a stressful lifestyle does not promote weight loss. If you think about it, our body already has a period of biological fasting that is the sleep phase, at night when we sleep we do not eat and we are "fasting" for even 12 hours.

Supplements?

You may wonder if it is right to take food supplements even though you are eating healthy food. Why do doctors often say that supplements are useless or can cause damage? The reason is that they do not know the subject; they reason by macro deficiencies and do not recognize that there are chronic micro deficiencies.

They are not considered as important pathologies but are sufficient to slow down the metabolism. The foods we eat, although healthy, do not always satisfy the daily needs of all the substances needed by our body. Also consider that today's foods are not the same as the food that our grandparents ate. If our goal is a longer and better quality of life then we need to integrate our intake, especially if we do physical activity.

We have established that it is necessary to do physical activity to reactivate or speed up our metabolism. With regards sporting activities we can divide the supplements into two categories. The first is for physical performance during which we expose the body to stress, the other for recovery which is the most neglected aspect.

For performance we can take branched-chain amino acids that nourish the muscle quickly by skipping the hepatic passage. Another supplement is creatine, a useful substance in some sports where a workout requires power and strength. For the recovery phase whey proteins can be taken as well as glutamine which is an amino acid with two roles, that of regulating the intestine to function properly and an immunostimulator. Finally, phosphatidylserine which is useful in lowering cortisol which increases performance and if it does not decrease it does not allow it to re-enter the anabolic phase.

These are natural substances that are safe for the body which your doctor will never prescribe for you because he does not understand the subject.

Conclusion

At the end of this brief journey, you have understood that the goal of physical fitness does not need to be achieved by following the classic "diet". Getting back in shape can be summarized in a few simple tips:

- Increase your basal metabolism by constantly training with weights. Start gradually and opt for all activities with high and interval intensity (HIT), rather than those with constant and prolonged intensity (aerobics);

- Have 5 meals a day: breakfast, snack, lunch, snack, dinner. Make breakfast a complete meal without including "sugary foods". Eliminate sugars and eat more vegetables respecting the balanced association of macronutrients. In the evening, do not eat carbohydrates except potatoes.

I wish you a good start so that you can experience what Hippocrates said *"that food is your medicine and that medicine is your food"*.

Warning

This book is about the personal experience of success in becoming physically fit. The information in this book is for cultural and educational purposes only and is not a medical prescription. The contents must not be understood as indications for a diet and it is advised to contact a specialist, in the presence of specific problems, like dysfunctions and intolerances. People who want to use the information described will do so under their own exclusive responsibility.